ABDOMINAL PAIN

UNDERSTANDING THE POSSIBILITIES OF CURING ABDOMINAL PAINS FOR GOOD

DR. J. SIMON

Contents

INTRODUCTION

Similar to an uninvited guest, abdominal pain can vary in severity from a minor annoyance to a major disturbance. It basically refers to any pain or discomfort you experience in the abdomen, which is the region between your chest and pelvis. Now, identifying this pain can be as difficult as playing hide-and-seek. It may come from the stomach, liver, gallbladder, intestines, or even the muscles, among other organs.

Abdominal pain can also come in a variety of forms, ranging from dull and cramping to sharp and stabbing. It's as though your body is using it to throw you a mystery book, and you're the investigator attempting to piece together the story.

The surprising part is that the antagonist in this tale isn't always stomach ache. Sometimes it's just a clue, your body's way of communicating in Morse code that something is off inside.

It's a challenging puzzle that frequently requires the assistance of a healthcare Sherlock to solve. Therefore, keep in mind the following when playing detective with stomach pain: pay attention to your body, pay attention to any signs, and seek professional advice whenever in doubt.

CHAPTER ONE

An Abdominal Anatomy

Imagine that your abdomen serves as the focal point of a busy city, with different organs contributing to the smooth operation of the show.

Stomach: Since the stomach is our own personal food processor, let's start there. Your meal is broken down into a semi-liquid consistency as it is mixed and churned.

Liver: The multifunctional marvel of the body is located right next door. It aids in digestion, generates vital proteins, and detoxifies. It's comparable to the stomach's superhero.

Gallbladder: The gallbladder is a tiny but important organ that is often found close by. When you eat something greasy, it stores the bile that the liver produces and releases it to aid in the breakdown of fats.

Pancreas: The pancreas, which regulates blood sugar, prowls about behind the stomach. It releases enzymes that aid in digestion and produces insulin to regulate blood sugar levels.

Small Intestine: The small intestine is the true workhorse of digestion, and it is located further south. It takes in the nutrients from the food and discards the less beneficial ingredients.

Large Intestine (Colon): The large intestine, also known as the colon, is reached after more descent. This is where electrolytes and water are absorbed, transforming the remaining material into the well-known waste form.

Kidneys: Well, they aren't quite in the abdomen, but they are adjacent. Urine is produced by the kidneys filtering your blood, eliminating waste and extra fluid.

Appendix: The appendix is tucked away in the lower right corner. It's similar to the little mystery in the abdomen; its exact function is unknown to us, but you'll know when it malfunctions.

Bladder: Your individual urine storage space is located right at the bottom. It has a talent for indicating when a pit stop is necessary.

That's it, a quick overview of the busy metropolis that is your stomach. Every organ plays a distinct part, and when they blend together, it resembles a dance with a tight choreography. If there are any disturbances, though, you may end up with that tricky stomach ache we previously discussed!

Common Reasons for Pain in the Abdomen

Ah, the great enigma that is abdominal pain. Numerous things can contribute to it, and each one has a unique role to play in the overall drama of discomfort. Let's investigate a few usual suspects:

Constipation, gas, and indigestion are examples of digestive shenanigans. Ingesting too much spicy food or neglecting to drink enough water can cause your digestive system to act out.

Infections: Abdominal pain may result from bacteria, viruses, or parasites choosing to establish a home in your digestive system. It's similar to an unwelcome guest staying longer than they should.

Inflammation: A number of illnesses, including appendicitis, gastritis, and inflammatory bowel diseases (such as Crohn's and ulcerative colitis), can lead to internal inflammation, which in turn can cause pain.

Gallstones: Visualize your gallbladder being overrun by tiny stones. It's what gallstones accomplish. They may result in sudden, severe pain, particularly after a high-fat meal.

Kidney stones: As they pass through your urinary tract, these tiny troublemakers can cause unbearable pain. It's less enjoyable than passing a rock concert.

Menstrual Pain: Women, this list does not apply to you. Abdominal discomfort from menstrual cramps can be comparable to a mini-tornado.

Ulcers: Eroding the protective lining of your digestive tract can cause ulcers in your stomach or duodenum, which cause a burning feeling.

Hernias: An organ that decides to play hide-and-seek in an inappropriate place can cause you to develop a hernia. It resembles an awkward attempt at contortion by your body.

Anxiety and Stress: Your body and mind work together dynamically. Tension and pain in your abdomen can be physical manifestations of stress and anxiety. It feels like your gut is having a little party due to your emotions.

Recall that this is merely a preview of the rogue's gallery of reasons for stomach pain. You should always seek professional medical advice if the pain is severe or feels like it's trying out for a major role in your life.

signs and symptoms

Symptoms and indicators frequently accompany abdominal pain, providing you with some indications as to what may be wrong. This is your decoder ring for understanding the language of tummy pain:

Type of Pain: Is it more of a dull, cramping ache or a sharp, stabbing pain? Sometimes the underlying cause of a pain can be inferred from its type.

Location: Where is the pain felt? Certain organs or problems can be indicated by diffcrent parts of the abdomen. upper abdomen? The liver and stomach may be giving out distress signals. lower abdomen? The focus may be on the reproductive system, the bladder, or the intestines.

Duration: Will this be a one-time appearance or a regular feature? Pain that is flecting may not be a serious concern, but persistent or recurring pain may be.

Intensity: Pain can be rated as "barely noticeable" to "I feel like I've been hit by a truck," and this rating system can help determine how serious a pain is.

Associated Symptoms: It is rare for abdominal pain to occur by itself. Watch out for symptoms such as fever, constipation, diarrhea, vomiting, nausea, and changes in bowel habits. These sidekicks can offer insightful knowledge.

Timing: Is the pain related to meals, occurring after eating, or waking you up in the middle of the night? Timing matters and can offer clues about digestive issues.

Bloating and Swelling: If your abdomen feels like it's hosting a balloon party or suddenly resembles a watermelon, bloating and swelling are telling you something's amiss.

Changes in Urination: Discomfort during urination or changes in frequency can point towards issues with the urinary system.

Fever: A fever accompanying abdominal pain could indicate an infection, and your body's heating up to fight the invaders.

Changes in Bowel Movements: Whether it's constipation, diarrhea, or unusual colors and textures, your bathroom habits might be trying to convey a message.

Remember, your body has its own Morse code, and these signs and symptoms are its way of sending distress signals. If the pain persists or becomes a recurring character in your life, it's time to play detective and consult with a healthcare professional.

CHAPTER TWO

Diagnosis and Assessment

When it comes to solving the mystery of abdominal pain, the process involves a bit of Sherlock Holmes detective work from your healthcare team. Here's a peek into the investigation process:

Medical History: Your doctor will kick things off by playing 20 questions. They'll ask about your symptoms, how long you've been experiencing them, and if there are any specific triggers or patterns.

Physical Examination: Get ready for a hands-on approach. Your healthcare detective will feel around your abdomen, checking for tenderness, swelling, or any unusual bumps.

Blood Tests: Time to draw some blood. Blood tests can help detect signs of infection, inflammation, or issues with your organs. It's like the body's version of leaving breadcrumbs.

Imaging Studies: X-rays, CT scans, or ultrasounds might be summoned to take a closer look at what's happening inside. It's like getting a backstage pass to the abdominal concert.

Endoscopy: If the situation calls for it, a tiny camera on a flexible tube might be sent on a reconnaissance mission down your throat or through other openings to inspect your digestive tract. It's the ultimate inside scoop.

Stool and Urine Tests: Sometimes, your bodily excretions hold valuable clues. Stool and urine tests can provide information about your digestive and urinary systems.

Diagnostic Procedures: Your doctor might recommend specific tests like a colonoscopy, upper endoscopy, or imaging of the gallbladder to get a more detailed picture.

Pregnancy Test: For the detectives with an extra chapter in their mystery novel, a pregnancy test might be in order. Sometimes, abdominal pain has a little surprise twist.

Laparoscopy: In some cases, a surgeon might make a small incision and use a camera to directly observe your abdominal organs. It's like a VIP tour of the inner workings.

Techniques for Counseling

Once the detectives have cracked the case and identified the culprit behind your abdominal pain, it's time to talk treatment strategies. Here's a diverse arsenal that healthcare professionals might deploy:

Medication Magic: Depending on the root cause, medications can work wonders. Antacids for indigestion, antibiotics for infections, or anti-inflammatory drugs for conditions like Crohn's disease—they're like the superheroes swooping in to save the day.

Dietary Adjustments: Sometimes, your diet needs a makeover. Cutting back on spicy foods, greasy delights, or lactose might be on the menu. It's like giving your digestive system a spa day.

Lifestyle Tweaks: Stress management techniques, regular exercise, and maintaining a healthy lifestyle can be key players in keeping abdominal pain at bay. It's like creating a peaceful environment for your internal organs.

Physical Therapy: For certain conditions, especially those involving the muscles and joints, physical therapy can be a game-changer. It's like sending in a team of specialists to restore balance.

Surgery: In more serious cases, when the abdominal pain is due to issues like gallstones, appendicitis, or hernias, surgical intervention might be necessary. It's the grand finale, where the surgeons take center stage.

Antibiotics: If the culprit is a bacterial infection, a round of antibiotics might be prescribed. It's like sending in the cavalry to defeat the invaders.

Probiotics: For digestive issues, introducing good bacteria through probiotics can help restore balance in your gut. It's like recruiting friendly forces to maintain peace.

Pain Management: Sometimes, pain relief medications might be used to ease the discomfort while addressing the underlying cause. It's like hitting the mute button on the pain symphony.

Remember, the treatment plan is as unique as the individual experiencing abdominal pain. What works for one might not be the magic potion for another. Your healthcare team will tailor their approach based on the specific diagnosis and your individual needs.

And just like any good detective story, communication is key. Keep the dialogue open with your healthcare professionals, and together, you can script a plan to bid farewell to abdominal pain and welcome in a new chapter of well-being.

When it comes to giving your abdomen some TLC at home, think of it as a self-care spa day for your insides. Here are some gentle remedies and practices that might help ease abdominal discomfort:

Stay Hydrated: Water is the unsung hero of many health issues. It helps with digestion and keeps things flowing smoothly. Sip on water throughout the day, especially if your abdominal pain is accompanied by diarrhea.

Peppermint Tea: A warm cup of peppermint tea can work wonders for soothing an upset stomach. The menthol in peppermint has a calming effect on the digestive system.

Ginger: Ginger has anti-inflammatory properties and is known to ease nausea. Try ginger tea, ginger candies, or simply add fresh ginger to your meals.

Heat Therapy: A heating pad or a hot water bottle on your abdomen can provide comforting relief. It's like a cozy blanket for your insides.

Probiotics: Incorporating probiotic-rich foods like yogurt or fermented foods into your diet can help maintain a healthy balance of gut bacteria.

Low-FODMAP Diet: If you suspect certain foods trigger your abdominal pain, consider trying a low-FODMAP diet. It temporarily reduces specific types of carbohydrates that can be hard to digest.

Avoid Trigger Foods: Keep an eye on what you eat. Spicy, greasy, or dairy-heavy foods might be the culprits, so give them a temporary vacation from your menu.

Relaxation Techniques: Stress and anxiety can amplify abdominal pain. Practice relaxation techniques such as deep breathing, meditation, or yoga to create a calm environment for your gut.

Over-the-Counter Medications: Antacids or medications containing simethicone can help alleviate gas and indigestion. Always follow the recommended dosage and check with your healthcare provider if you have any concerns.

Rest: Sometimes, all your body needs is a bit of downtime. Ensure you're getting enough sleep and listen to your body's signals to take it easy when needed.

Remember, these home remedies are like gentle whispers of care for your abdomen. However, if your symptoms persist, worsen, or if you're unsure about the cause of your abdominal pain, it's crucial to consult with a healthcare professional. They can provide personalized guidance based on your specific situation.

Emotional Health and Coping Mechanisms

Abdominal pain doesn't just take a toll on your physical well-being; it can also play mind games with your emotions. Here are some coping strategies to navigate the emotional rollercoaster that often comes with abdominal discomfort:

Mindful Breathing: Practice deep, mindful breathing to help manage stress and anxiety. Inhale slowly, hold for a moment, and exhale gently. It's like giving your mind a mini-vacation.

Distraction Techniques: Engage in activities that divert your attention away from the pain. Whether it's reading, listening to music, or watching a favorite show, distraction can be a powerful ally.

Positive Visualization: Picture yourself in a serene place. It could be a peaceful beach, a calming forest, or your favorite cozy spot. Visualization can help create a mental escape from the discomfort.

Seek Support: Don't be afraid to lean on friends, family, or a support group. Sharing your experience and feelings can be therapeutic, and you might find comfort in knowing you're not alone.

Therapeutic Techniques: Consider exploring therapeutic techniques like cognitive-behavioral therapy (CBT) or relaxation therapy. These can provide tools to manage stress and improve overall emotional well-being.

Set Realistic Goals: On days when the pain is more prominent, set achievable goals for yourself. Celebrate small victories, and don't be too hard on yourself if you need to take it easy.

Mind-Body Practices: Incorporate mind-body practices like yoga or tai chi into your routine. These can promote relaxation, improve flexibility, and enhance your overall sense of well-being.

Educate Yourself: Knowledge is power. Learn more about your condition and the factors that contribute to your abdominal pain. Understanding can empower you to make informed decisions about your health.

Stay Positive: Maintain a positive mindset. Focus on the aspects of your life that bring joy and fulfillment. Positivity can be a strong ally in facing challenges.

Mindfulness Meditation: Practice mindfulness meditation to stay present in the moment. It can help you accept and navigate the challenges with a calmer perspective.

Remember, it's okay to acknowledge and express your emotions. Coping with abdominal pain is not just about physical resilience; it's a holistic approach that includes your emotional and mental well-being. If the emotional impact becomes overwhelming, consider reaching out to a mental health professional for additional support. You're not just managing abdominal pain; you're taking care of your whole self.

Red Flags and When to Seek Medical Attention

While some abdominal pain might feel like a passing inconvenience, certain red flags warrant immediate attention from the healthcare squad. Here are some signs that it's time to hit the panic button and seek medical help:

Severe Pain: If your abdominal pain is so intense that it feels like a WWE smackdown in your gut, don't brush it off. Severe pain could indicate a serious underlying issue.

Sudden and Intense Pain: A sudden onset of severe pain might be a red flag. It could be related to conditions like appendicitis or a kidney stone, which often come with a "surprise attack" vibe.

Pain with Vomiting: If your abdominal pain is accompanied by persistent vomiting or the inability to keep anything down, it's time to summon the healthcare cavalry.

Persistent Pain: If the pain persists for an extended period, especially if it's getting worse rather than better, it's a sign to consult with a healthcare professional.

Pain after Injury or Trauma: If your abdominal pain follows an injury or trauma to the abdomen, seeking medical attention is crucial. It could indicate internal damage.

Bloody Stool or Vomit: When your bodily excretions start resembling a crime scene, it's a clear signal to get medical help. Bloody stool or vomit can be associated with serious conditions.

Difficulty Breathing: Abdominal pain paired with difficulty breathing could point to a more critical issue. It's a red flag that requires immediate attention.

Pain during Pregnancy: If you're pregnant and experiencing abdominal pain, especially if it's accompanied by other symptoms like bleeding, it's crucial to seek prompt medical advice.

Signs of Infection: Fever, chills, and signs of infection along with abdominal pain could indicate a more systemic issue that needs urgent attention.

Previous Abdominal Surgery: If you've had abdominal surgery in the past and are experiencing new or worsening pain, it's essential to get it checked out.

Remember, your body has its own alarm system, and these red flags are like the sirens going off. Don't hesitate to seek medical attention if you notice any of these warning signs—it's better to be safe than sorry. The healthcare professionals are there to unravel the mystery and ensure your well-being.

CHAPTER THREE

Abdominal Pain in Special Populations

Abdominal pain doesn't discriminate; it can make an appearance in various populations, each with its own set of considerations. Let's take a quick look at how abdominal pain plays out in different groups:

Children and Adolescents: Kids can be little mysteries when it comes to expressing discomfort. Abdominal pain in this group could be due to various factors like infections, constipation, or even emotional stress. It's essential to pay attention to any changes in behavior and seek medical advice if the pain persists.

Pregnant Individuals: Ah, the joys of pregnancy! Abdominal discomfort during pregnancy is not uncommon and can be attributed to the expanding uterus, hormonal changes, or digestive issues. However, if the pain is severe, persistent, or accompanied by other concerning symptoms, it's crucial to consult with a healthcare provider.

Elderly Population: Abdominal pain in the elderly can be tricky to diagnose as it might be related to age-related changes, medications, or underlying health conditions. It's essential for older individuals to communicate any discomfort to their healthcare provider for a thorough evaluation.

Individuals with Chronic Conditions (e.g., IBS, Crohn's Disease): Those dealing with chronic conditions like irritable bowel syndrome (IBS) or Crohn's disease often have a more complex relationship with abdominal pain. Management may involve a combination of medications, lifestyle changes, and regular monitoring.

Individuals with Diabetes: Abdominal pain in individuals with diabetes can be linked to various factors, including gastrointestinal complications, nerve damage, or fluctuations in blood sugar levels. Maintaining stable blood sugar levels and addressing any digestive issues is crucial.

People with Mental Health Conditions: Emotional well-being is closely connected to abdominal health. Individuals with mental health conditions, such as anxiety or depression, may experience abdominal pain as a physical manifestation of their emotional state. A holistic approach that addresses both mental and physical health is often necessary.

Individuals with Neurological Disorders (e.g., Parkinson's Disease): Neurological conditions can influence the digestive system and contribute to abdominal pain. Individuals with conditions like Parkinson's disease may experience gastrointestinal symptoms that require careful management.

Cancer Patients: Abdominal pain in cancer patients can result from the disease itself, side effects of treatment, or complications. It's crucial for cancer patients to communicate any new or worsening pain to their healthcare team for proper evaluation and management.

In each of these special populations, a personalized and multidisciplinary approach is often necessary. Healthcare providers consider the unique characteristics and needs of each group to develop effective strategies for managing and addressing abdominal pain. If you or someone you know falls into one of these categories and experiences abdominal discomfort, consulting with a healthcare professional is the best course of action.

Conclusion

Abdominal pain, the elusive visitor to the core of our being, is a signal that our body uses to communicate distress. It's not just a standalone discomfort; it's a narrative that unfolds differently for each individual. From the mundane to the serious, abdominal pain can be a puzzle that requires careful deciphering.

Understanding the anatomy of the abdomen is like having a map for this intricate landscape. The stomach, liver, gallbladder, intestines, and their companions play their roles in a delicate dance of digestion and function. Yet, when this harmony is disrupted, abdominal pain steps into the spotlight.

Diagnosing the source of abdominal pain is akin to detective work. Medical history, physical examinations, blood tests, and imaging studies form the toolkit for unraveling the mystery. It's a journey that may lead to dietary adjustments, medications, or even surgical interventions.

But beyond the physical realm, abdominal pain takes a toll on our emotional well-being. Coping strategies, mindfulness, and seeking support become essential components of the holistic approach to well-being.

Abdominal pain doesn't discriminate; it touches various populations differently. Children, pregnant individuals, the elderly, those with chronic conditions, or individuals with mental health concerns all navigate a unique landscape of abdominal discomfort.

In conclusion, abdominal pain is a multifaceted experience that requires attention, understanding, and collaboration between individuals and their healthcare providers. Whether it's a passing discomfort or a persistent challenge, the journey to relief involves a blend of medical expertise, self-care, and a touch of resilience. So, if you find yourself in the midst of an abdominal tale, remember that you're not alone, and the narrative can evolve into one of well-being with the right guidance and care.

THE END